Survival Medicine for Beginners

A Quick start Guide to Coping with Injury during Disaster

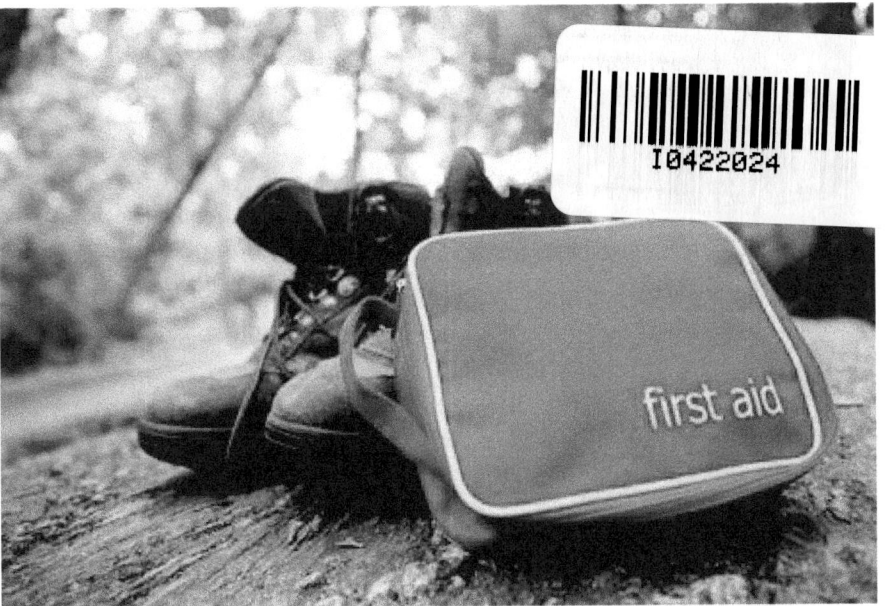

Prepping and Survival Series

M. Usman

Mendon Cottage Books

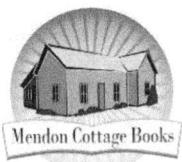

JD-Biz Publishing

Disclaimer

The information is this book is provided for informational purposes only. It is not intended to be used and medical advice or a substitute for proper medical treatment by a qualified health care provider. The information is believed to be accurate as presented based on research by the author.

The contents have not been evaluated by the U.S. Food and Drug Administration or any other Government or Health Organization and the contents in this book are not to be used to treat cure or prevent disease.

The author or publisher is not responsible for the use or safety of any diet, procedure or treatment mentioned in this book. The author or publisher is not responsible for errors or omissions that may exist.

Warning

The Book is for informational purposes only and before taking on any diet, treatment or medical procedure, it is recommended to consult with your primary health care provider.

Our books are available at

1. Amazon.com
2. Barnes and Noble
3. Itunes
4. Kobo
5. Smashwords
6. Google Play Books

Table of Contents

Introduction

Disaster can strike at any given moment – whether you live in close proximity to natural hazards such as an earthquake zone or active volcano, or whether you live in a seemingly safe urban area. Your geographical location is a major factor when considering the different ways that you may be exposed to dangers, however this is an issue that has the potential to affect you at home, on holiday, or even when you're visiting a new area. In such situations, it may be difficult to reach the emergency services or contact someone that may be able to help you – you could find yourself isolated from human settlement and left to your instinctive devices.

The basics to survival medicine are often overlooked and cast aside when it comes to common knowledge. How many of us could use indigenous plants as an antiseptic? How many of us could bind a wound using natural dressings? These are key skills that we have no use for in our everyday lives and of course, we can always use a helpful app or the internet to help us, right? But, what could we do in situations when those luxuries are out of reach and the only tools we have is the environment around us?

This guide will cover the essential basics in survival medicine, giving you a basic knowledge and understanding of how to cope with injuries in such distressing situations. From the contents of your survival pack to using potentially life-saving plants and applying emergency techniques – this guide will help you to build up a solid foundation. If you ever find yourself injured in a disaster situation, you'll know where to begin.

Chapter 1 – What's In Your Kit?

I – The Basic contents of a good first aid kit

Carrying the essential medicine and first aid supplies can be a life-saving action. You'll need a waterproof bag with multiple sections and pockets that is large enough to accommodate all of your supplies. Choose a bag with a bright color for ease of visibility. Here is a checklist of the basics that should be packed within your first aid kit:

✓ Report Cards and Waterproof Markers (for making note of any injuries).

✓ Pocket knife (folding blades are preferable for saving space)

✓ 7 day supply of any prescription medicine that you or any family members take

✓ Latex or Vinyl Gloves

✓ Large Safety Pins (at least a dozen)

✓ A Roll of Adhesive Cloth and Plastic Tape

✓ Roller and Triangular Bandages (Cravat)

✓ A Range of Waterproof Plasters (varied sizes are preferable)

✓ Sterile Gauze Pads (4x4 and 8x10") and Cotton Swabs

✓ Sterile Water and Mild Disinfectant

✓ Antibiotic Solution and Anti-Diarrheal Medicine

✓ Clothesline (can be used as rope or for pressure binding)

✓   Aspirin or Tylenol

✓   A thick stack of sanitary napkins or adult nappies

✓   Small Pair of Scissors

II – Conditions for use and precautions

The list given on the previous page is a guide and is by no means extensive. Depending on your situation and geographical location, more specific medicines may be more appropriate.

In terms of the medicines found within your pack, read any labels and instructions carefully before use and ensure that all bottles or tablets are labeled clearly and correctly. Follow any dosage instructions particularly carefully and make note of the times or number of doses you or a family member has taken. If you or any family members have any allergies, be particularly careful in the administration of medication and dressings. Whether this is latex gloves or a particular painkiller, ensure these allergies are written in the notebook or on the report cards that should always be found within your kit. Never use any expired medical products and replace your medicine supply every six months.

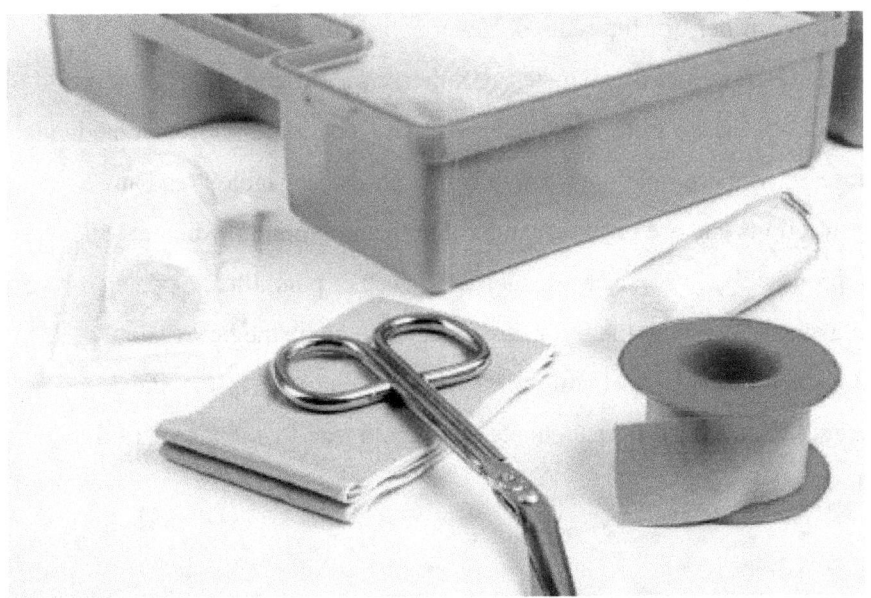

Before using any blade or scissors in a medical procedure, ensure that they are sterilized either by flame or with a disinfectant. This prevents any further infection or contamination of the wounded area. Prior to using your kit, be comfortable with its entire contents and the multiple uses each piece may have. For example, sanitary napkins and adult nappies can be incredibly useful for pressure bindings and controlling blood loss.

III – Alternative methods for when your pack is not enough

If a situation arises in which your current supplies are depleted, make use of any similar items in your pack such as using gauze pads for binding or multiple layers of roller bandages in the creation of a pressure pad. Use your supplies sparingly and always pack plenty of spares when it comes to plasters and dressing materials. Items such as wound dressings should never be reused due to their direct contact with the injury. However, binding cloth used on sprains or dislocations can always be washed and dried using sterilized water, for future uses. Never contaminate your first aid kit with used dressings and waste material, rather store these items separately and dispose of them carefully in the appropriate location. In terms of medicinal doses, if you are running low in a particular drug or tablet, read any instructions that are provided and ration the remaining medicine appropriately. In some cases, such as the use of painkillers, spacing out your intake and reserving them for dire situations can be the best option. However, in the case of antibiotics you should always follow the doses as suggested, because an inadequate dose could lead to a longer period of illness or infection.

Chapter 2 – Maintaining Your Health

I – Retaining fluids and preventing dehydration

Having a reliable first aid kit is essential for making it through tough disaster scenarios. However, maintaining your health in general can prevent further complications later down the line. The first aspect of your health that you should address in a disaster situation is water. Retaining fluids in a hot climate can be especially difficult, so ensure that you are out of the sun during the peak afternoon hours and that you travel in as much shade as possible. Keeping out of the direct sunlight will reduce your perspiration rates and consequently reduce your water loss. If you have access to long-sleeved clothing or a hat, be sure to wear them when out of shaded areas. If you don't have these luxuries, minimize your exposure time and use any materials you have available to you to prevent yourself from over-heating. If you're in a colder climate, water can be just as scarce and is still vital for your body to continue functioning as normal. Once again, keep yourself covered and protected from the cold and prevent dehydration.

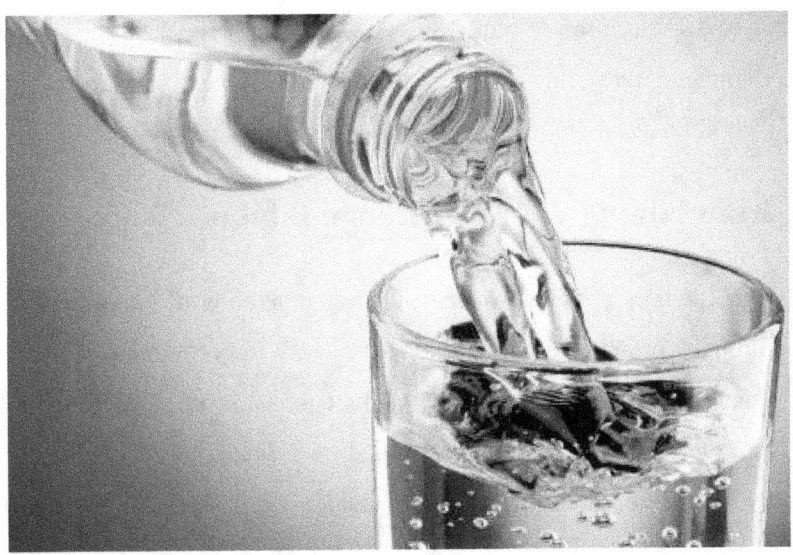

Here are a number of other steps that should be followed in order to prevent dehydration:

- Limit the time you spend carrying out vigorous or sweat inducing activities (if you're in a relatively safe location, there is no need to travel further and the closer you remain to your original area, the more likely you are to receive aid).

- Drink water reservedly when consuming food. Your body utilizes water during digestion, so always drink a small amount of water with any food that you eat.

- If you have not located a reliable source of water, ration your supplies carefully and consider the need for emergency uses too. This is essential if you are stranded or isolated and don't have direct access to aid or a settlement with a mains supply.

- Control your breathing. This may seem like an odd point to arise, however in the stressful event of disaster, panic attacks and anxiety are, of course, more likely to have an effect on you. These reactions can result in raised blood pressure and even hyperventilation – in the long term, this leads to a greater consumption of energy and the body's water supply, in respiration and perspiration.

II – Maintaining your nutritional intake

Although not as essential as water, your food intake is still important in maintaining your health and preventing illness. Without regular and nutritional food intake, your physical and mental capacity will decrease, leading to potential lapses in judgment and poor decision making. Food supplies should be packed within a survival kit and include dried foods with a long shelf-life and high energy content. This may include items such as cereal and protein bars. Aside from high energy foods, foods with high water content, such as fruits, berries, and vegetables are essential and carry a wealth of important vitamins and minerals. Depending on your location, you may be able to utilize fruits and berries from your environment. However, you should only ever consume wild foods such as these if you are completely certain of their appearance and in situations of great need. Incorrectly identifying wild foods and mistaking them for another species can be incredibly dangerous and even fatal in some circumstances. On a similar note to conserving your water supplies, ensure that any food supplies are rationed appropriately and that they are stored safely, away from insects, pests, and animals. Always store your food and water separately in order to reduce the chances of spoilage.

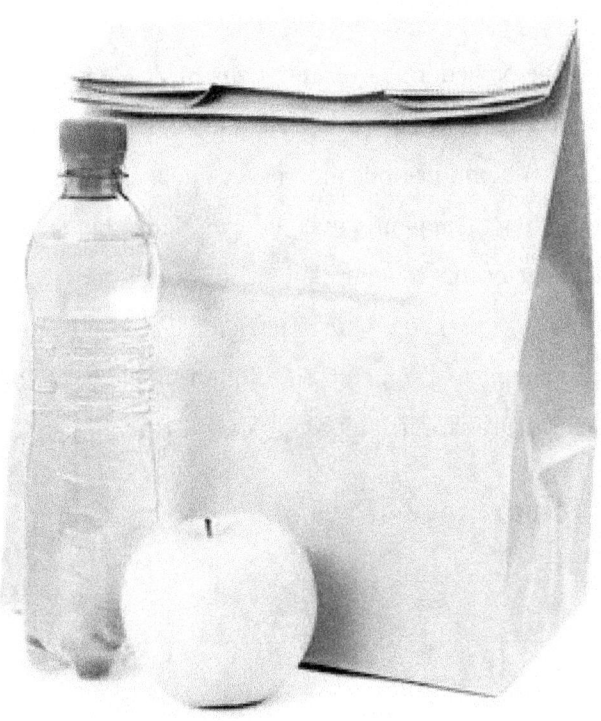

III – A guide to sterile and safe hygiene practices

Maintaining a high standard of personal and practical hygiene is essential for preventing disease or infection in any disaster or emergency situation. Following simple steps such as washing your hands before tending to wounds or handling food should not be overlooked and in a survival scenario, as these practices can be life-saving.

Keeping a positive state of personal hygiene will not only benefit your health, but also reduce your chances of harboring any infections or insect-related illness. Showering daily is a good place to start, although this relies upon your access to safe water. In situations where conventional bathing is not possible, exposing your skin to the sun for at least sixty minutes can also cleanse your body. Caution should be taken in order to prevent sunburn from occurring.

In terms of sterile procedure, never reuse any blades, pins, needles, or materials that have previously been used to tend to a wound or injury, as this can induce further complications in terms of infection. Metal objects can be sterilized by heating them gently over an open flame, but take care that no melting or damage occurs to your blade whilst this is carried out. Mild disinfectants that are packed within your first aid kit can be used to sterilize equipment and any instruction on their dilution should be followed carefully in order to reduce any skin irritations or adverse reactions.

IV – The importance of rest

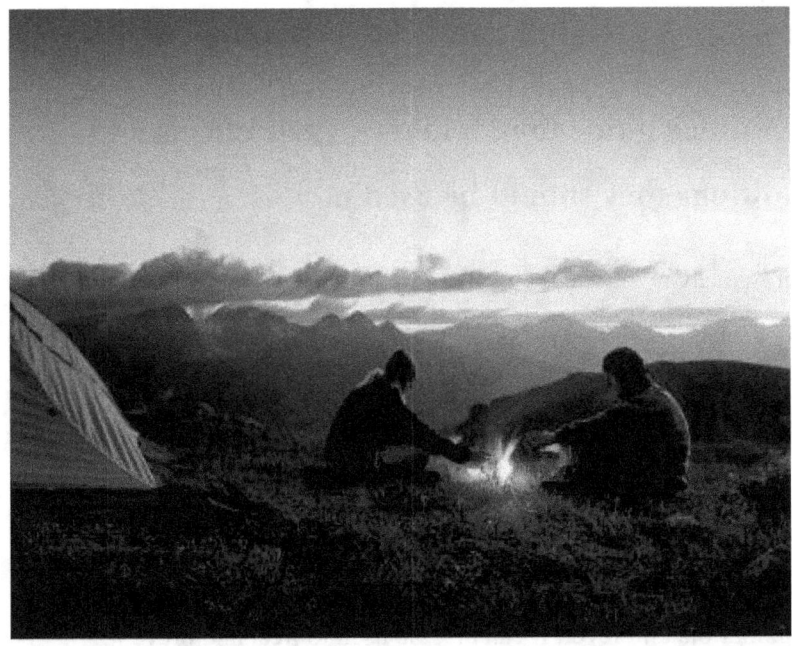

Resting your body under the stressful events of disaster can be incredibly difficult; however this basic need should never be cast aside. Considering the high likelihood that your water and nutritional intake will be lower than it should be, rest is even more essential. Moreover, it gives your body time to naturally repair, so in terms of maintaining your health, it is vital. If travelling, you should take an average of approximately fifteen minutes of rest for every hour of physical activity that you are engaged in. This range will vary depending on your physical fitness and terrain. When resting, ensure that you are out of the sun and protected from any changes in temperature that may occur during the night. As hard as it may seem, find ways to make yourself comfortable, whether this is using additional clothing or vegetation as a pillow or covering yourself in an emergency blanket that should be included in your survival pack. Take as much rest as your body needs and never push your body to exhaustion. Your survival depends on the ways in which you use your energy.

Chapter 3 – Using medicines from your kit

I – A quick guide to painkillers, their effects and conditions they should be used in

As previously mentioned, your first aid kit or survival pack should include a number of conventional 'over the counter' medicines, one of which should be a painkiller. Aspirin is a common drug that can be packed into your kit and used in a number of situations. This drug can be used to reduce fever and inflammation, both of which could have been induced by an insect bite or sting or an allergic reaction. Aspirin works by reducing the chemicals in your body (such as histamine) that are produced to cause pain, inflammation, and fever. It can also be used to treat and prevent cardiovascular related conditions. However, this should only be carried out in the presence and under the supervision of a trained doctor. You should not use aspirin to treat any condition if you have sustained any recent intestinal or stomach bleeding.

You should take aspirin as directed on the instructions or label on the original packaging of the drug, and never take an incorrect dose as this may cause adverse effects on your body. If your bottle of aspirin has a strong scent of vinegar associated with it, do not use the drug – this is a sign that the medicine may have expired and is no longer effective. Once you have taken a dose of aspirin, make a note in your Medical Report Cards and include all relevant details such as the time and volume of your intake.

Another similar drug to aspirin is Tylenol. This medicine can act as another form of pain relief and for the reduction of fever symptoms. Tylenol is a versatile drug that can be used in the treatment of headaches, colds, toothaches, muscle ache and backache, or arthritis. Once again, when taking

Tylenol, you should follow any label or instructive material completely. Overdosing on this particular drug can lead to serious liver damage and even death - pay close attention with your doses and record any uses in the report cards. Never combine medications as this can lead to an incorrect dose and once again may have serious implications.

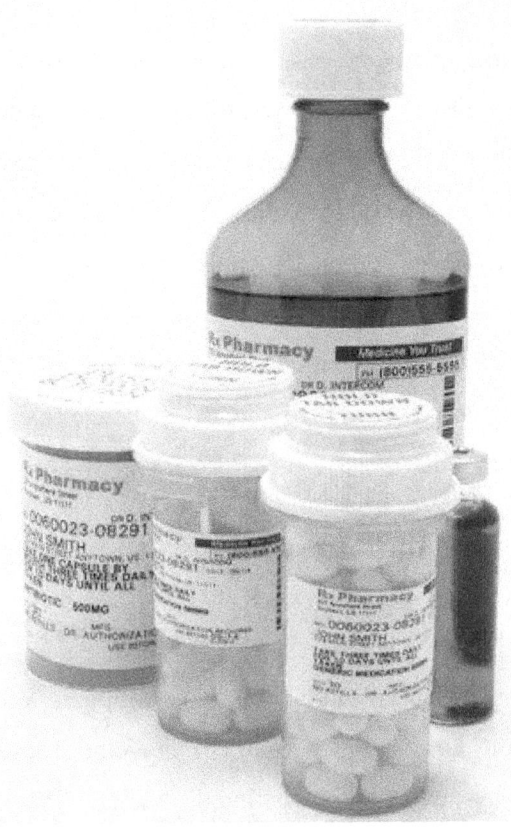

II – Antiseptics and their uses in preventing infection

Antiseptic medicines prevent the growth of pathogens (disease causing micro-organisms) and should be used to clean wounds after a rinsing of the area with sterile water. Antiseptics are used to kill bacteria upon rapid contact and are usually applied directly to the skin of people or animals.

Similarly, disinfectants also kill bacteria, however their difference is that they are usually applied to surfaces and non-living objects – they contain harsher chemicals that may not be as suitable to more sensitive skin. Always follow any dilution instructions when using disinfectants, as this is vitally important in avoiding any corrosive or harmful reactions when they come into contact with your skin.

Hydrogen peroxide and iodine based solutions can be used as antiseptics and can be applied to grazes, cuts, and wounds when cleaning the area. Disinfectants can also be used to sterilize any equipment that may be used in a surgical or wound addressing situation. You should never put equipment, or even your hands, in direct contact with an open wound – this can cause cross contamination and further infect the area. The gloves contained within your first aid kit should also be used when handling harsh, undiluted disinfectants such as hydrogen peroxide, to reduce the chances of a negative reaction with your skin.

III – Antibiotics and the situations they should be used in

In comparison to antiseptics and disinfectants, antibiotics are used to treat bacterial infections through the ingestion of medicine. These medicines can operate in two ways, either by preventing the bacteria from repairing any damaged DNA or by physically weakening the bacteria's cell wall until it reaches its limit and bursts. Bacterial infections can be contracted from a number of sources, with the most common being contaminated water. This can be through drinking unclean water or even bathing in it – ear infections are easily contracted in this way. When using a water source for any activity, ensure its cleanliness and boil or purify before use to kill any bacteria present.

Antibiotics are available by prescription and should always be taken as instructed, however they can also be purchased over the counter at a pharmacy. Penicillin is a common antibiotic that can be used to treat ailments such as ear infections. However you should ensure that you do not possess an allergy to this medication before taking it. Penicillin should also never be taken if you have serious asthma or any kidney and blood clotting disease.

Chapter 4 – Using indigenous plants that have medicinal properties

I – Identifying and using plants as painkillers

If a situation arises in which you have no access to your medical supplies or if your supplies have been exhausted, it can be extremely helpful to know how to make use of indigenous plant species and their uses for medicinal practice.

In terms of painkillers, aspirin itself is originally derived from the bark of the willow tree. Therefore the use of this plant can have the same effects as a conventional painkiller. A poultice (crushed leaves and plant matter used to treat a wound) of willow bark, dock leaves sorrel, or plantain can be used and applied to areas where you are experiencing pain, such as headaches or backache. Another method is to crush the leaves and if possible, add a little animal or vegetable fat to create a salve; this can be stored and used for future reapplication. Willow trees are easily identifiable by their sweeping branches and draping leaves and only fresh bark should be used in a medicinal practice – dead wood may contain micro-organisms and bacteria that could cause an infection.

Dock leaves are often used to relieve the pain of nettle or insect stings and are respectively located near outcrops of the nettle plant itself. They have broad leaves, often speckled with red and are usually the only other plants growing directly amongst the nettle bed. Once again, simply crushing and rubbing the leaf against the painful area can bring instant relief and a soothing sensation. However, this is not particularly a specific property of this plant species. The act of rubbing a leaf over a sting disperses the toxin or acid, reducing its effect. Any moisture from the leaf will also soothe the area. The use of dock leaves is an easy method to remember due to their widespread nature, distinctive appearance, and close proximity to a stinging species.

If the pain you are experiencing is overwhelming or you are in need of rest, a number of common plant species can also be used as a natural sedative. Once again, willow bark is amongst them, as well as elderflower and elm bark. For a sedative effect, these medicinal plants must be ingested, often in the form of a tea as this releases their oils and allows their relaxing properties to enter your system directly. This tea can be used to provide

relief from headaches and migraines.

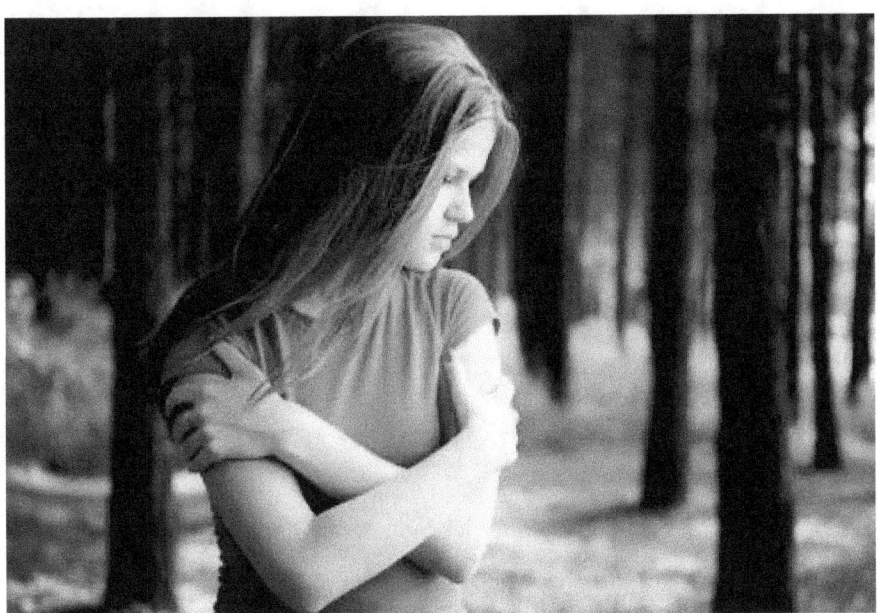

II – Common plants with antiseptic properties

In additional to pain relief and sedative effects, plants can also be used as a natural antiseptic. These medicinal plants can be used to cleanse wounds, sores, or rashes when conventional antiseptics or disinfectants are not available to you. The most common plants that can be used to cleanse wounds are wild onion and garlic. These are easily identifiable plants with a strong, characteristic scent that will reveal their location. As they require moist soils for growth, they are often located close to river and stream banks. Crushing the garlic or onion with a blade will release the juice that contains the antiseptic properties. Use a sterile bandage or gauze to soak in the juices and then apply to the wound. Once again, you can store the juices and the plants themselves for future use.

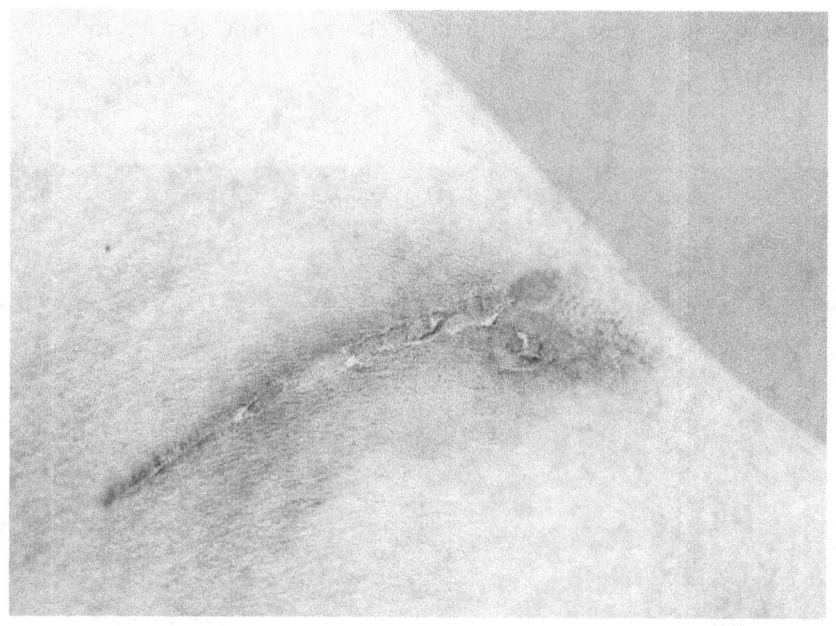

Other plants with antiseptic properties include the bark of the white oak tree (identifiable from its leaf shape and light bark color) and burdock root. These two plants can be used in conjunction to create a decoction (the boiling of plant matter to release its essential oils and medicinal chemicals into the water), which once again, can be applied to a wound in the cleansing procedure. Antiseptics should only ever be used externally and should never be ingested. When using plant matter for cleansing a wound, ensure that the leaves or bark itself is clean and dirt free, as the presence of bacteria can further infect the wound.

III – Precautions and dangers of using plants as medicines

You should only use plant material for medicinal purposes if you have no other conventional substances or drugs available to you. The identification of plant species can be incredibly difficult in a survival situation, due to stress and the varying terrain and environments you may find yourself in. Never use a plant species as a medicine unless you are certain of what it is and how it should be used. The strength of the chemicals within the plants will vary, so be particularly cautious when approximating doses and always apply a small volume of the salve or poultice first, to check for any adverse or allergic reactions. Never use dead plant material for any medicinal purpose, as decay and rot indicates the presence of bacteria and the ingestion or use of this plant may cause further problems for your health.

Plants can be dried by gently heating over a flame (when protected or wrapped within a damp material) or by the sun and stored in your survival pack for future usage. This increases the length of time they can be used for. Always label any medicinal plants that you store or carry with you and store different species separately. Plants used for medicinal or nutritional purposes should never be stored together, because this reduces the chances of them being used incorrectly and causing an adverse reaction.

Chapter 5 – Injuries to bones or joints

I – Methods for binding injuries

Damage caused to bones and joints can be incredibly painful and more difficult to care for compared to a cut or graze. The reasons for this are simple; your bones and joints control movement and without comprehensive attention, they may heal incorrectly and possibly even cause further damage such as internal bleeding.

When choosing a method to bind an injury you must first asses the size of the damaged area and how much support it will require. This may seem like an obvious statement however an injury such as a broken ankle would need a much higher degree of padding and protection compared to a broken arm. This is simply due to the amount of pressure that will be exerted upon it. The roller bandages contained within your first aid kit can be used for arm and wrist injuries and the triangle bandages for addressing particular joint areas with further support. Using a long length of bandage can be helpful for creating a sling in the event of a broken arm, however the bones itself should also be further bound with additional bandages and support. If bones set incorrectly, they can be incredibly painful, so never leave a broken bone unsupported. Tape can be used to tie any bindings that need to be made, as can rope or natural fibers. When binding an injury, ensure that the blood circulation is not being totally cut-off and if the area includes an open wound, ensure that the area is given time to breathe when you are stationary and preferable by a fire (there's less chance for a bacterial or insect infection by doing it this way).

II – Materials that can be used as dressings

When dressing a wound or injury you must first ensure the area has been disinfected and sterilized comprehensively. This can include the use of a pharmaceutical or natural antiseptic applied directly to the skin and a sterile, disinfected gauze pad that has been doused with an antibacterial solution. Dressings should be tight enough to prevent further infection however wounds will heal quicker if given air too. If travelling through rough, dirty and dangerous terrain, keeping all wounds covered completely. Ensure the material used as direct contact dressing is soft and doesn't cause any further irritation to the area. Bind the dressing with further support if needed and always finish the dressing with a waterproof layer. This may be in the form of a waterproof bandage or plaster. You may also use plant oils such as Aloe Vera to provide a further watertight barrier, preventing the chances of further infection.

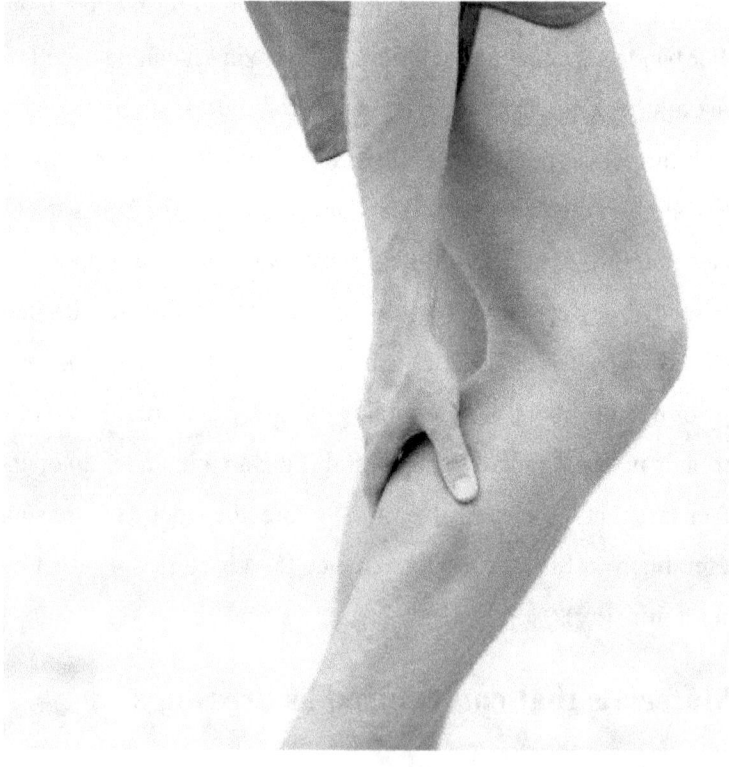

III – A guide to caring for dislocations and sprains

Dislocations are injuries that occur when a joint (such as the ball and socket shoulder joint) separates and displaces from its usually position. A sprain is another injury to a joint that occurs when the ligament tissue between the bones has been damaged. When caring for dislocations and sprains, you should reduce as much pressure as possible to the area and allow it as much rest as you are able to. Elevating the joint can help to reduce the swelling and inflammation to the area and also reduces the pressure, allowing a faster healing process. The conventional method for treating sprains is the RICE method, Rest (24 hours), Ice followed by heating, compression with padding or a splint and finally elevation. Most of this procedure can be carried out in a disaster situation, however in terms of a substitute for the ice, you may be able to utilize cold metal objects with the filling of cold water, as this will provide a level of relief to the area. Cold compresses using leaves or a damp cloth can also soothe the area. In terms of using a splint to align the joints, use young tree saplings, as they are strong and supple and combine the joint to another for the correct alignment.

Chapter 6 – Emergency and Lifesaving Techniques

I – Controlling blood flow from wounds

When it comes to open wounds in a disaster situation, controlling bleeding immediately is of the utmost importance. Replacing lost bodily fluids is not usually possible and so preventing further blood loss can be a lifesaving skill to possess. Applying direct pressure to the wound can be an extremely effective method to stem the blood flow and should be maintained for the entire period of time needed for the platelets within your blood to form a clot and seal the wound temporarily. Direct pressure should be applied with the use of a sterile dressing, preferably a bandage of generous length, which will provide layers of protection and support.

Following a period of approximately thirty minutes, if an open wound is still bleeding despite being held under direct pressure, you should apply a pressure dressing to the area. A pressure dressing is comprised of a thick sterile gauze pad and several layers of think roller bandages. The pressure binding should be tighter than the direct pressure dressing; however it should not be cutting off the blood circulation to the rest of the limb. When using a pressure binding, never remove the dressing even if the bandage becomes saturated, as this can cause a sudden revert in pressure and allow the blood to flow openly once again.

Once the pressure dressing has been in position for 2 days, you may begin to remove the layers of binding slowly to replace them with fresh dressings of a thinner composition. When changing the dressing of an open wound, always check the area comprehensively for any signs of potential infection and deal with this appropriately with an antiseptic. The wound should also be bathed periodically with sterile water in order to keep the area clean and free of micro-organisms.

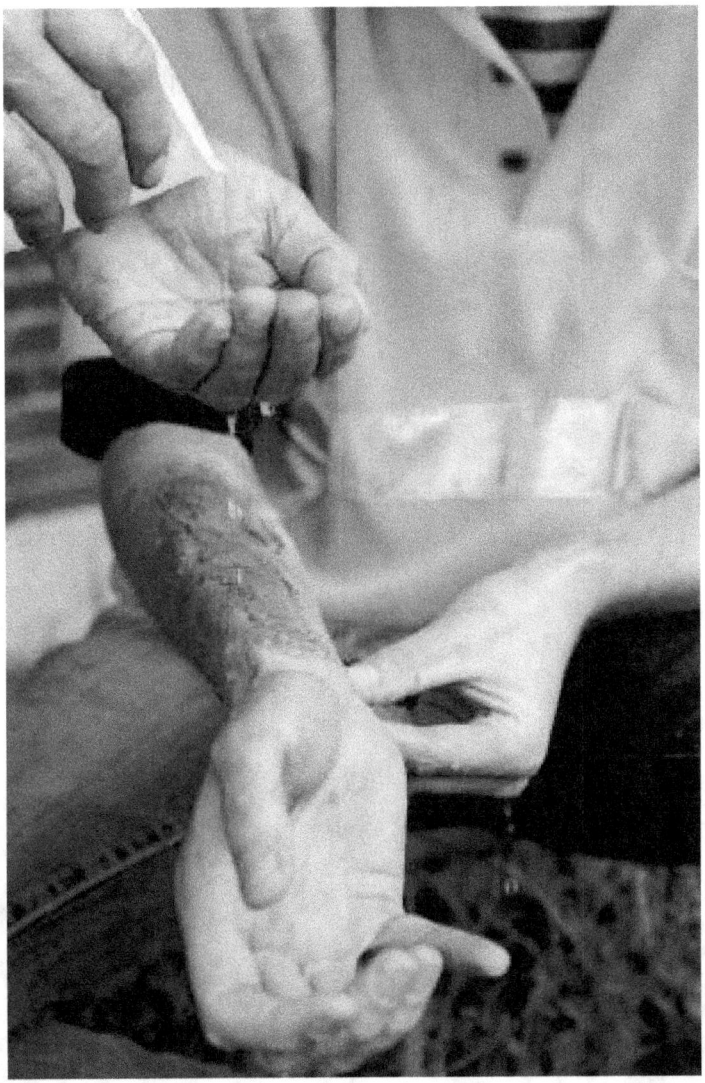

II – A quick guide to CPR

CPR is a process that artificially allows the body to breathe and pumps oxygen using a combination of compressions to the chest area and breathing directly into the patient's windpipe. Prior to performing CPR you should attempt to call for aid or send another person to look for a way to contact the emergency services. Once this has been completed, compose yourself and follow these next steps:

1. Check the victim for a response. Call their name. If you receive no response and the victim is not breathing or moving you should begin chest compressions.

2. Apply pressure to the centre of the chest by interlocking your hands into a fist and pressing down firmly to a depth of two inches. Repeat the compressions thirty times. Your pumping should correlate to a heartbeat of one hundred beats per minute.

3. In between sets of compression, tilt the head of the victim back and lift the chin to open their airways. Pinch their nose and blow air into their mouth until you see their chest rise in height. Supply two breaths to the victim, each lasting just one second.

4. Repeat the process of thirty compressions and two breaths until further aid arrives.

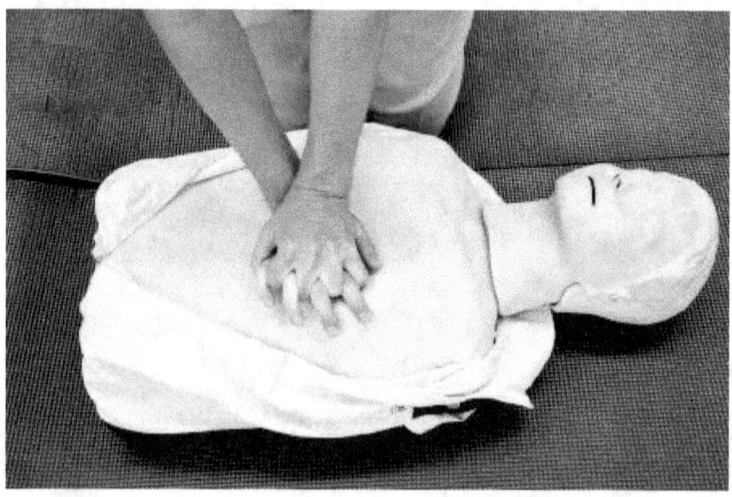

Conclusion

Disaster situations can be times of high stress, disorientation, and panic. Before attempting any medical procedure, always take a moment to compose yourself and take in your environment, the supplies available to you, and the time you have to carry out the medical process. Having read this guide you should feel a degree of relief in knowing a number of life-saving methods and practices that can be used in a survival situation. All of the information should be used as a guide only and if professional care is available, you should utilize this as soon as possible. From curing headaches with the aid of indigenous plants to binding a wound with a pressure dressing – you are now a step ahead on the road of survival medicine.

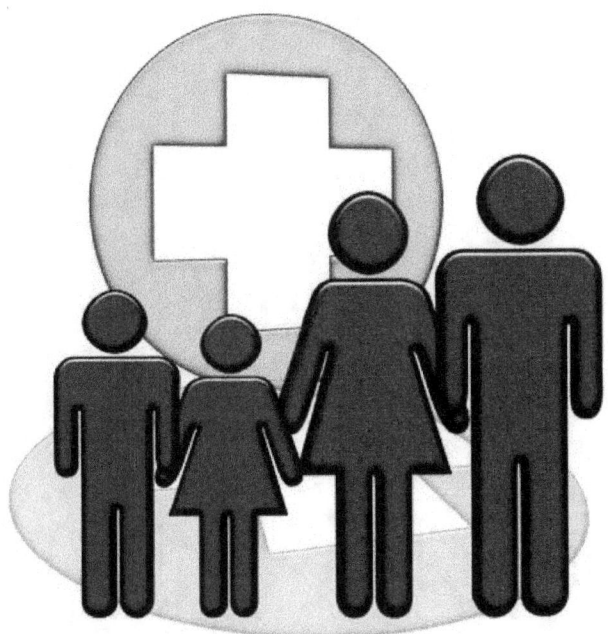

Author Bio

Muhammad Usman is a distinguished medical graduate of Allama Iqbal medical college (AIMC). He is a professional writer who has been in the field for more than 4 years. During this time he has produced 10,000+ articles, blogs and eBooks on various niches related to diseases, health, fitness, nutrition and well-being. He is a regular contributor to several journals related to medicine and surgery. He is the editor of several journals and newspapers.

Check out some of the other JD-Biz Publishing books
Gardening Series on Amazon

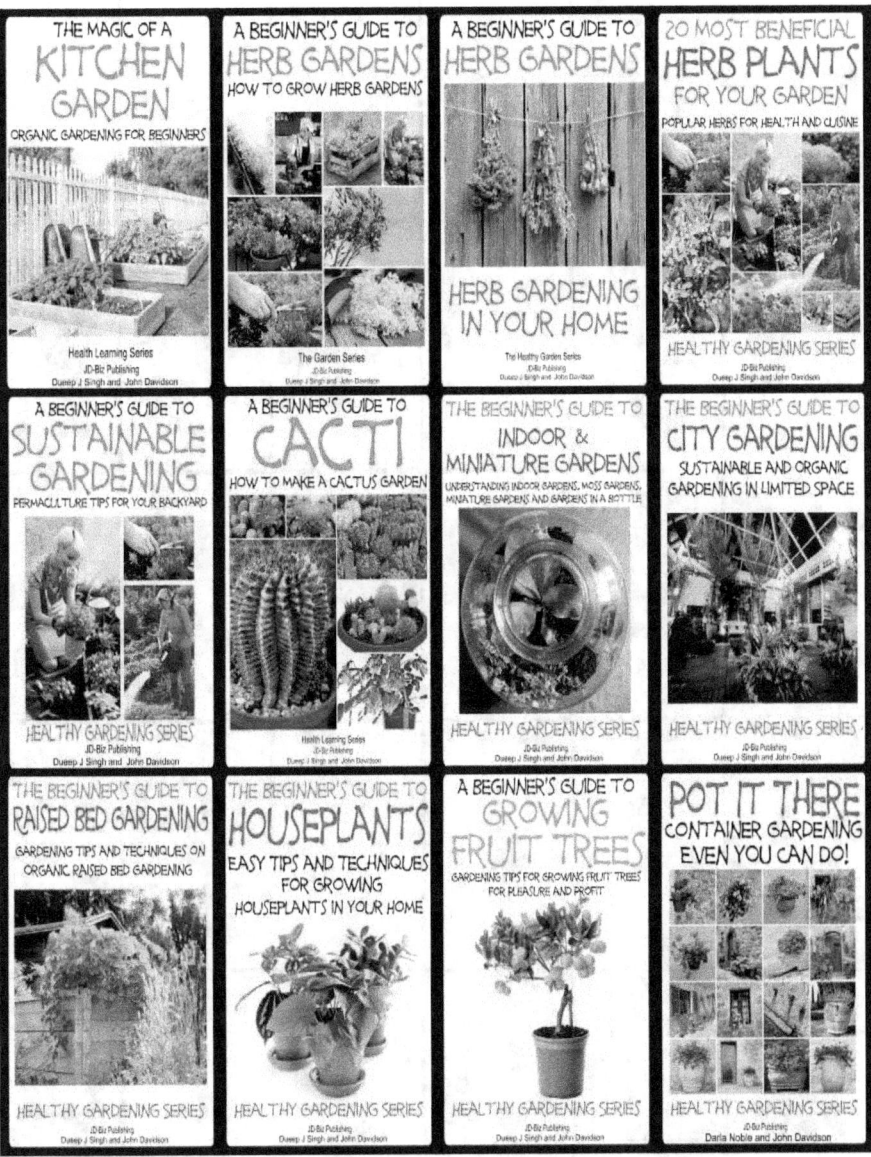

Health Learning Series

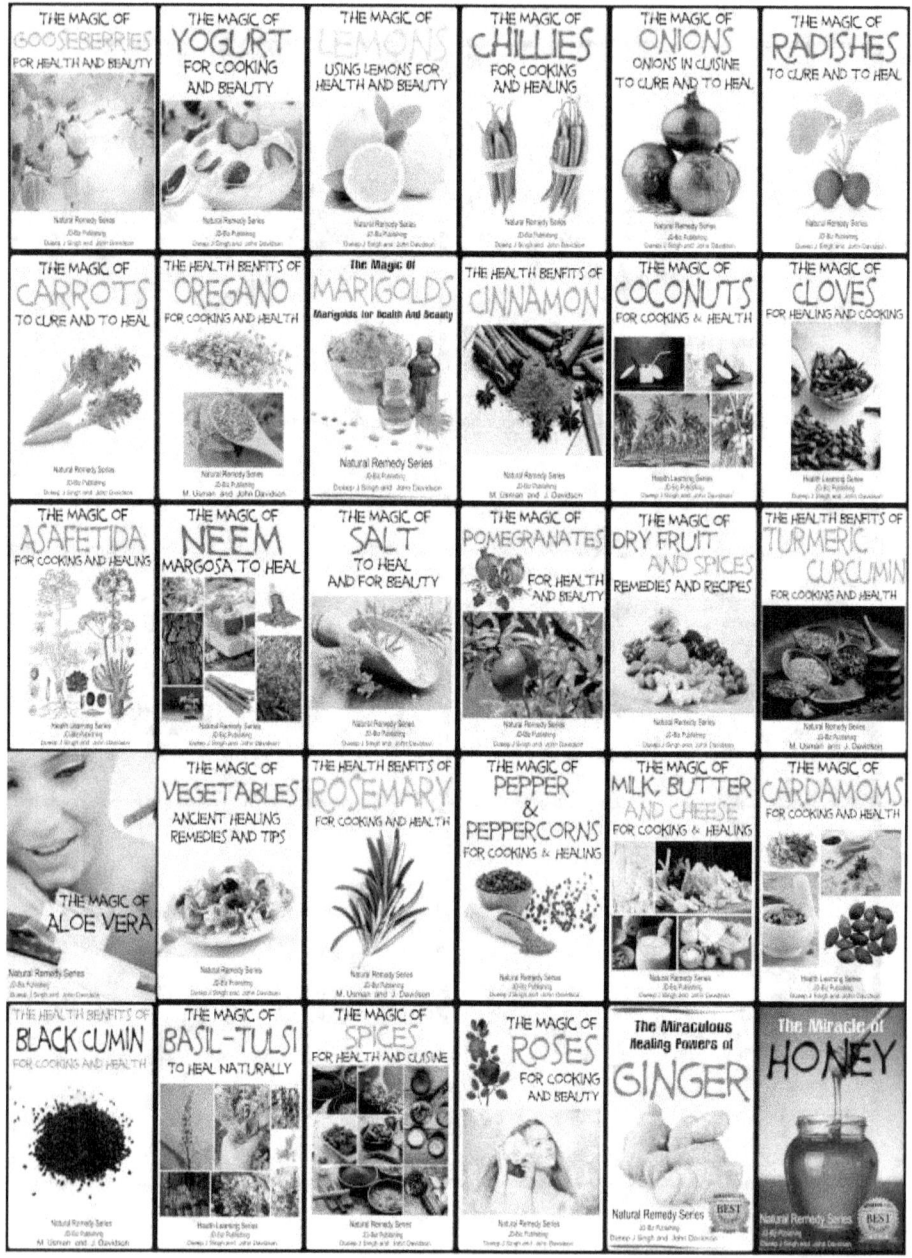

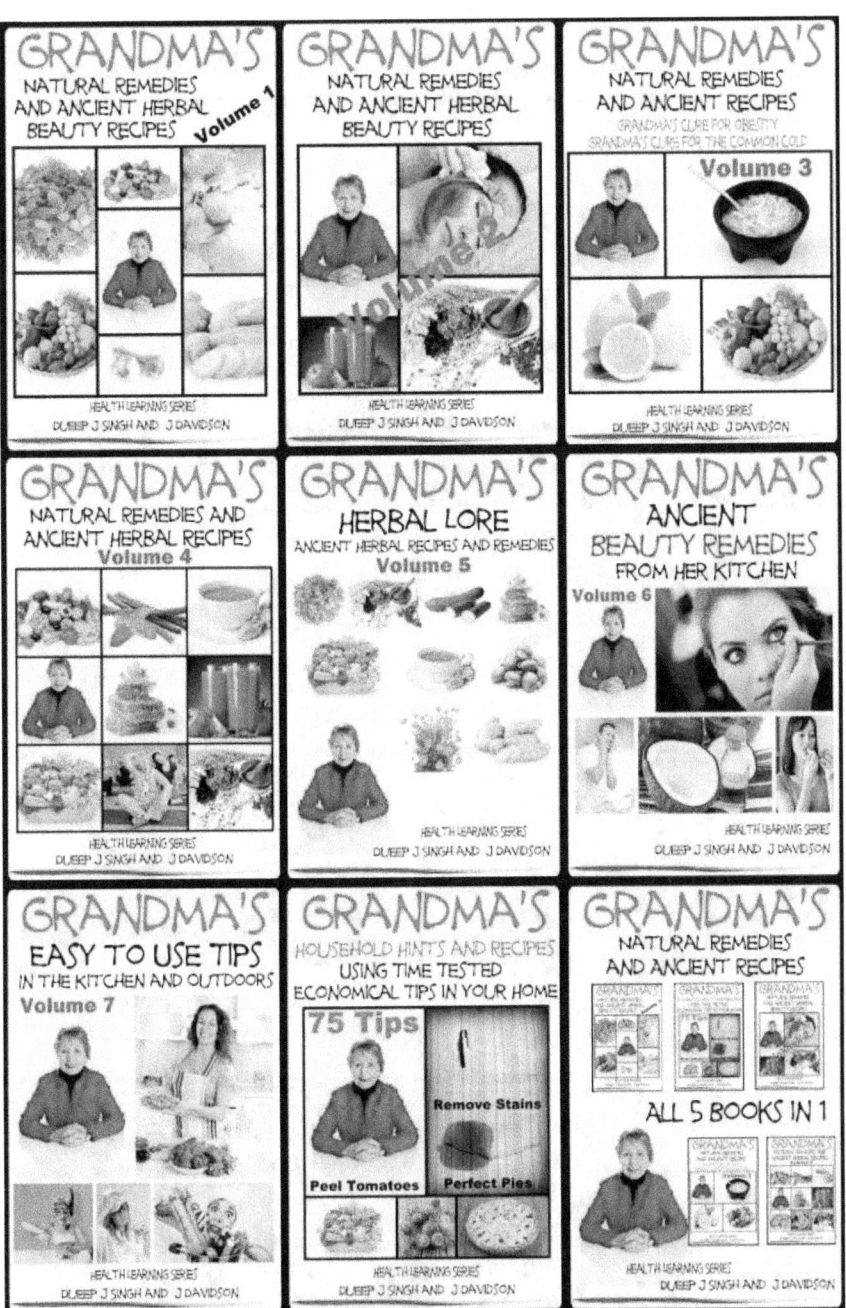

Country Life Books

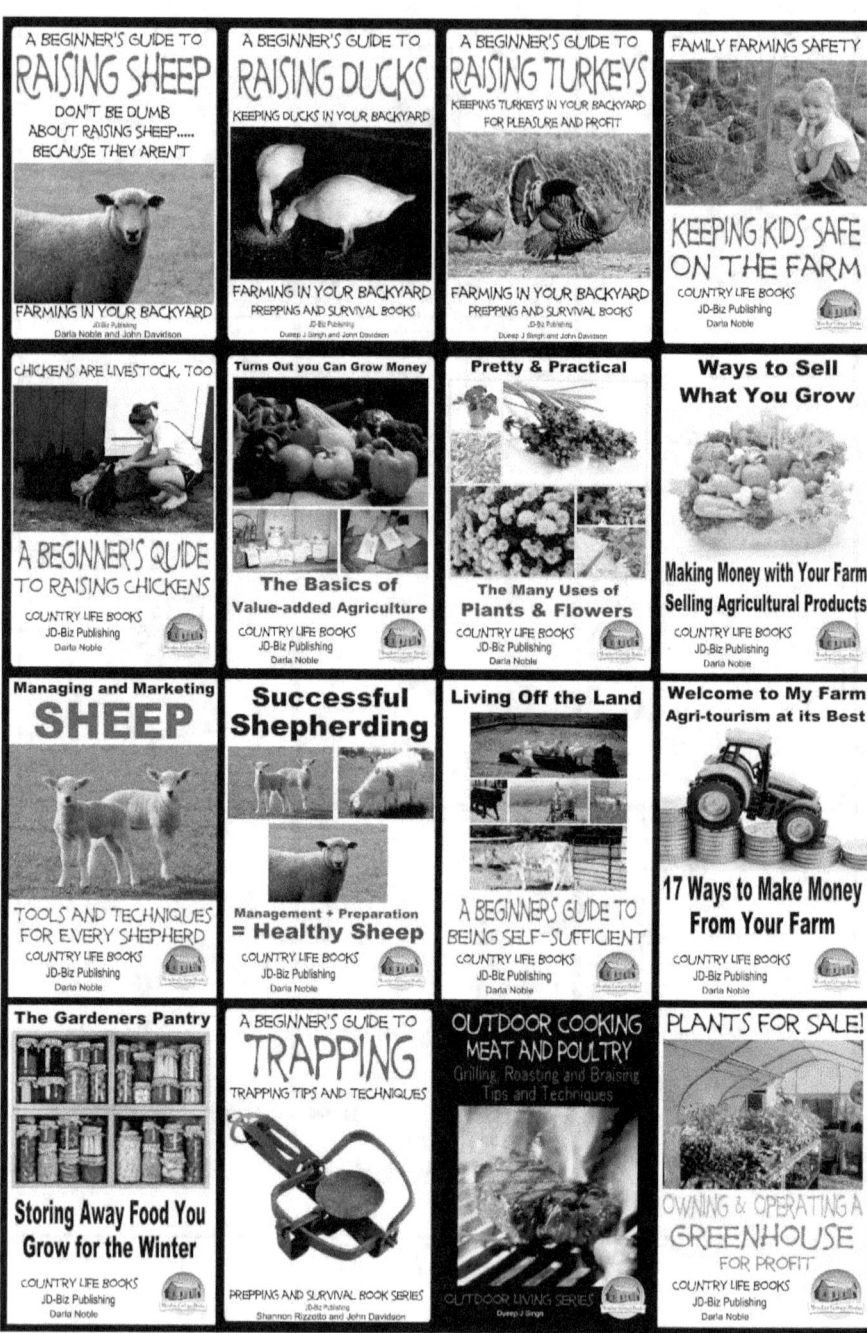

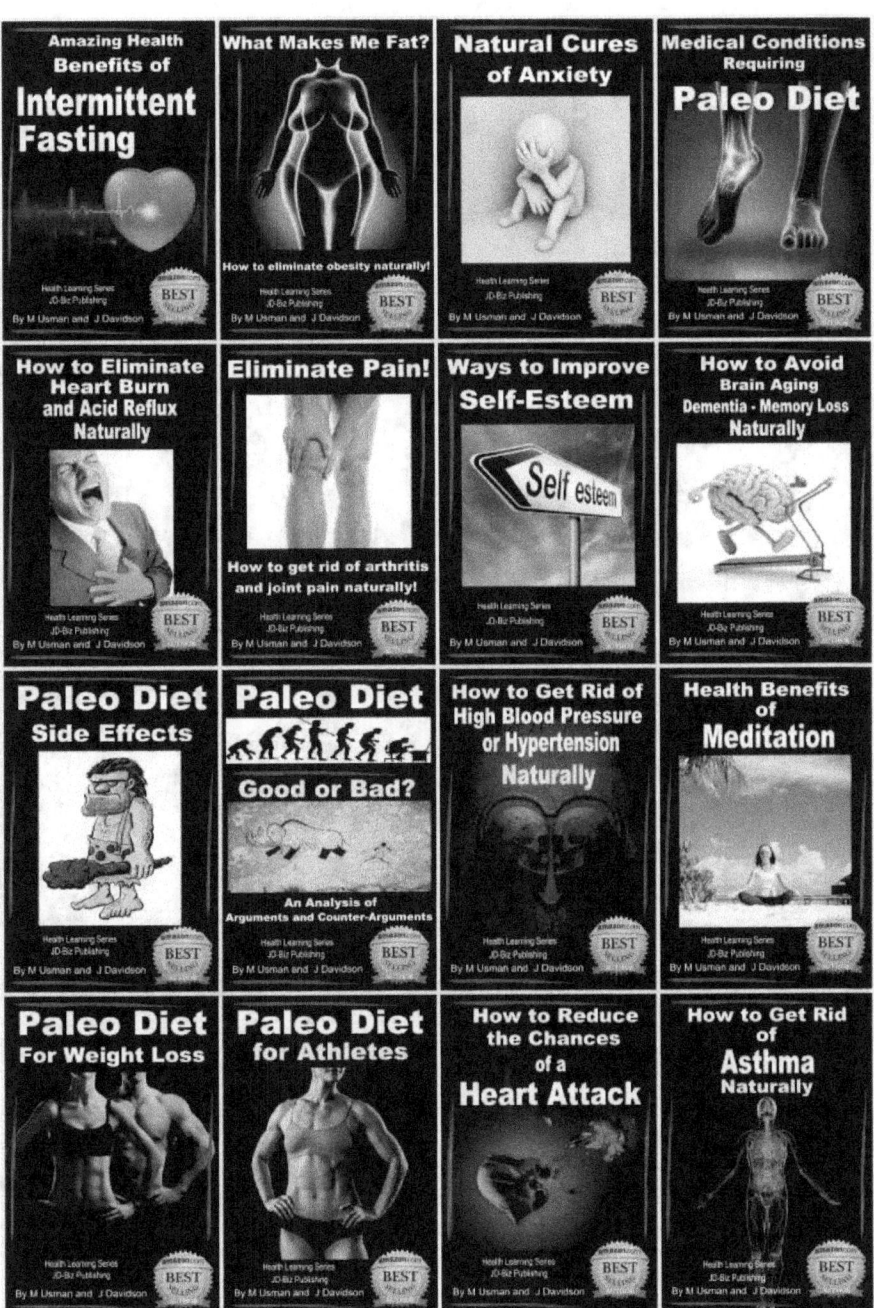

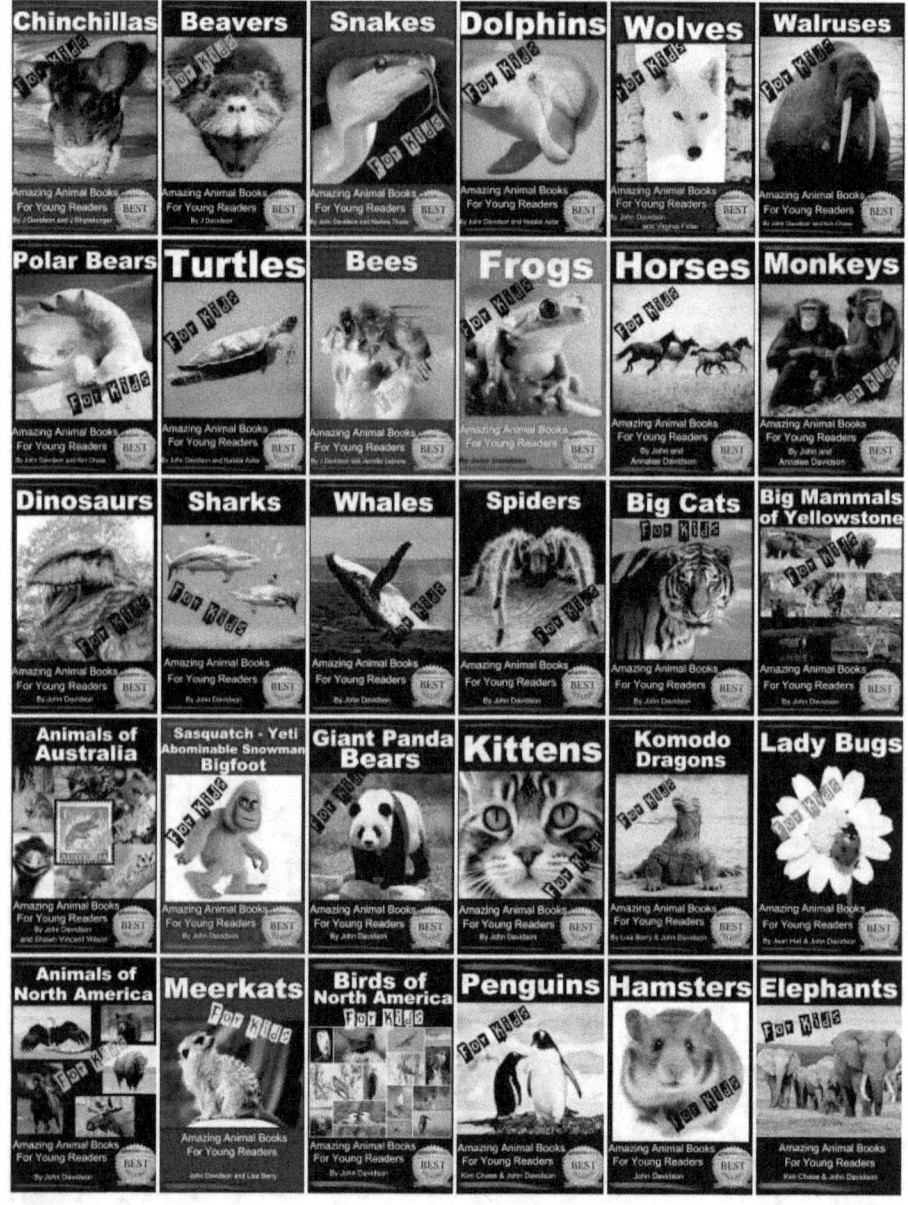

Learn To Draw Series

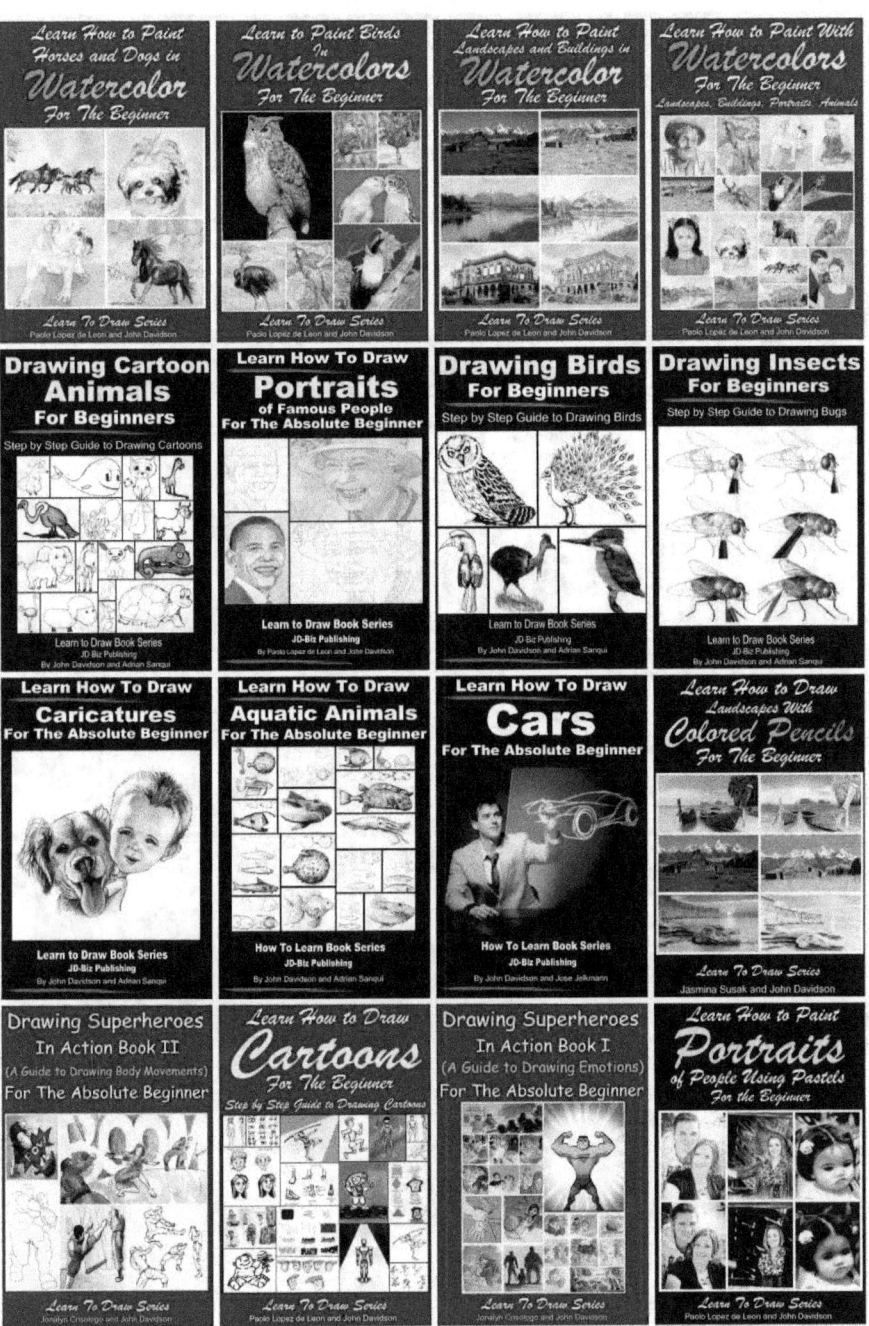

How to Build and Plan Books

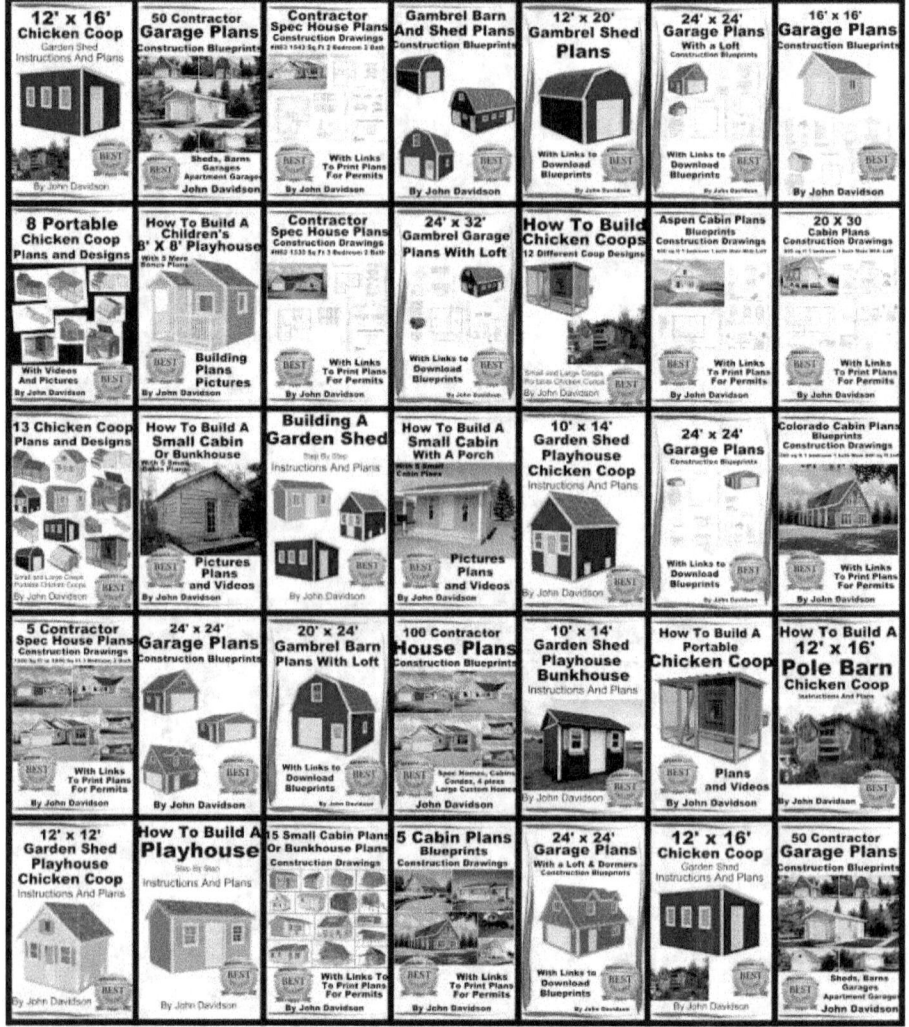

Entrepreneur Book Series

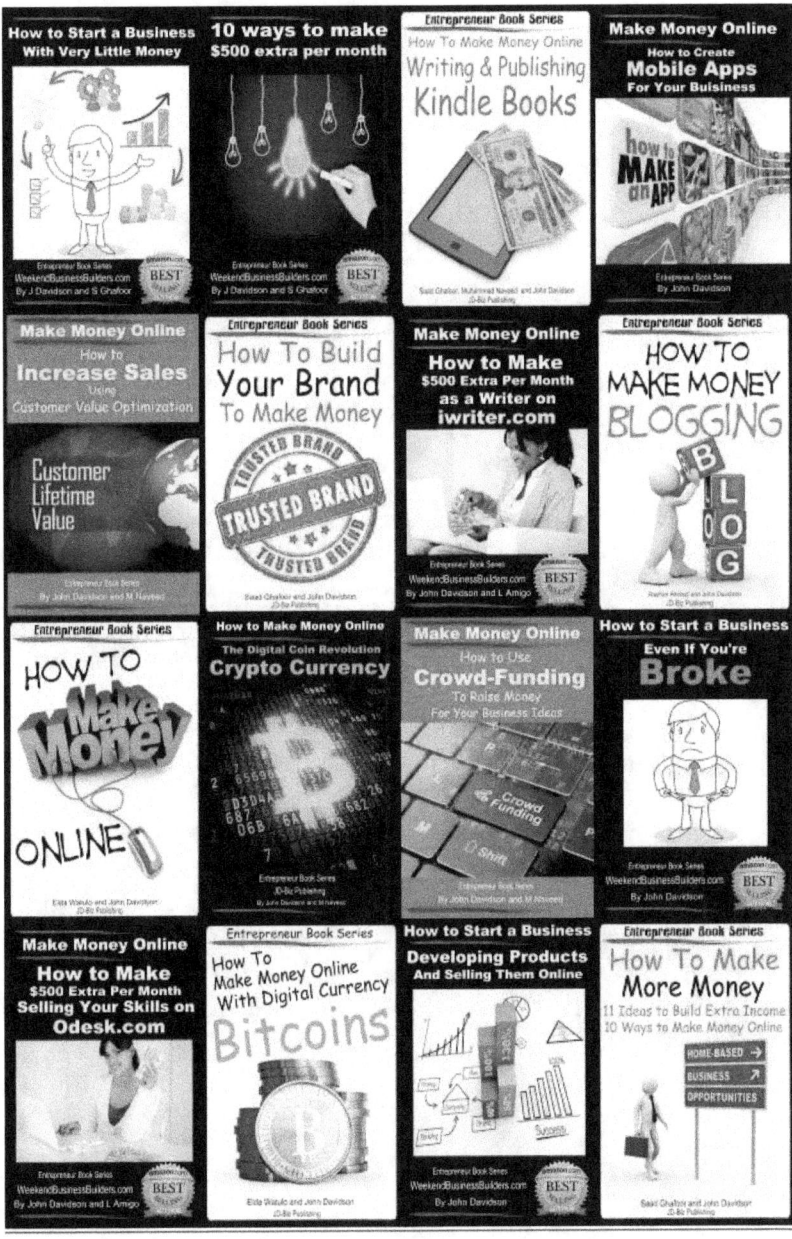

Our books are available at

1. Amazon.com

2. Barnes and Noble

3. Itunes

4. Kobo

5. Smashwords

6. Google Play Books

Publisher

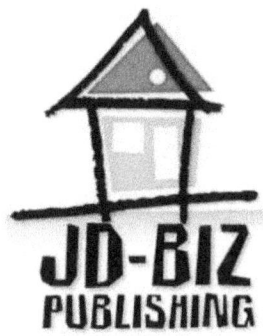

JD-Biz Corp

P O Box 374

Mendon, Utah 84325

http://www.jd-biz.com/

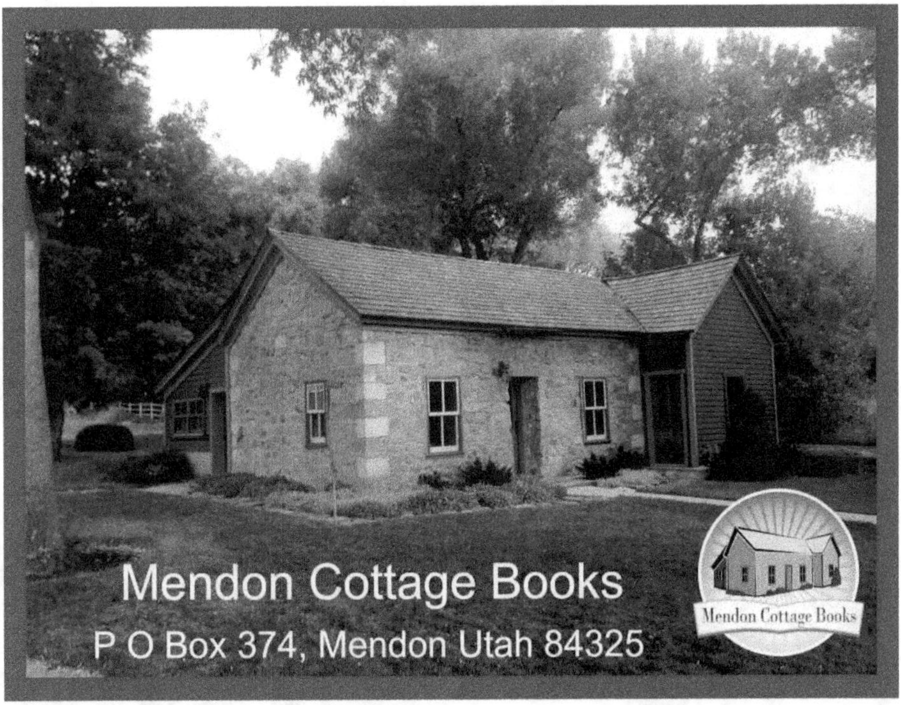

Mendon Cottage Books
P O Box 374, Mendon Utah 84325
Mendon Cottage Books